A'Quita's

Broken

Heart

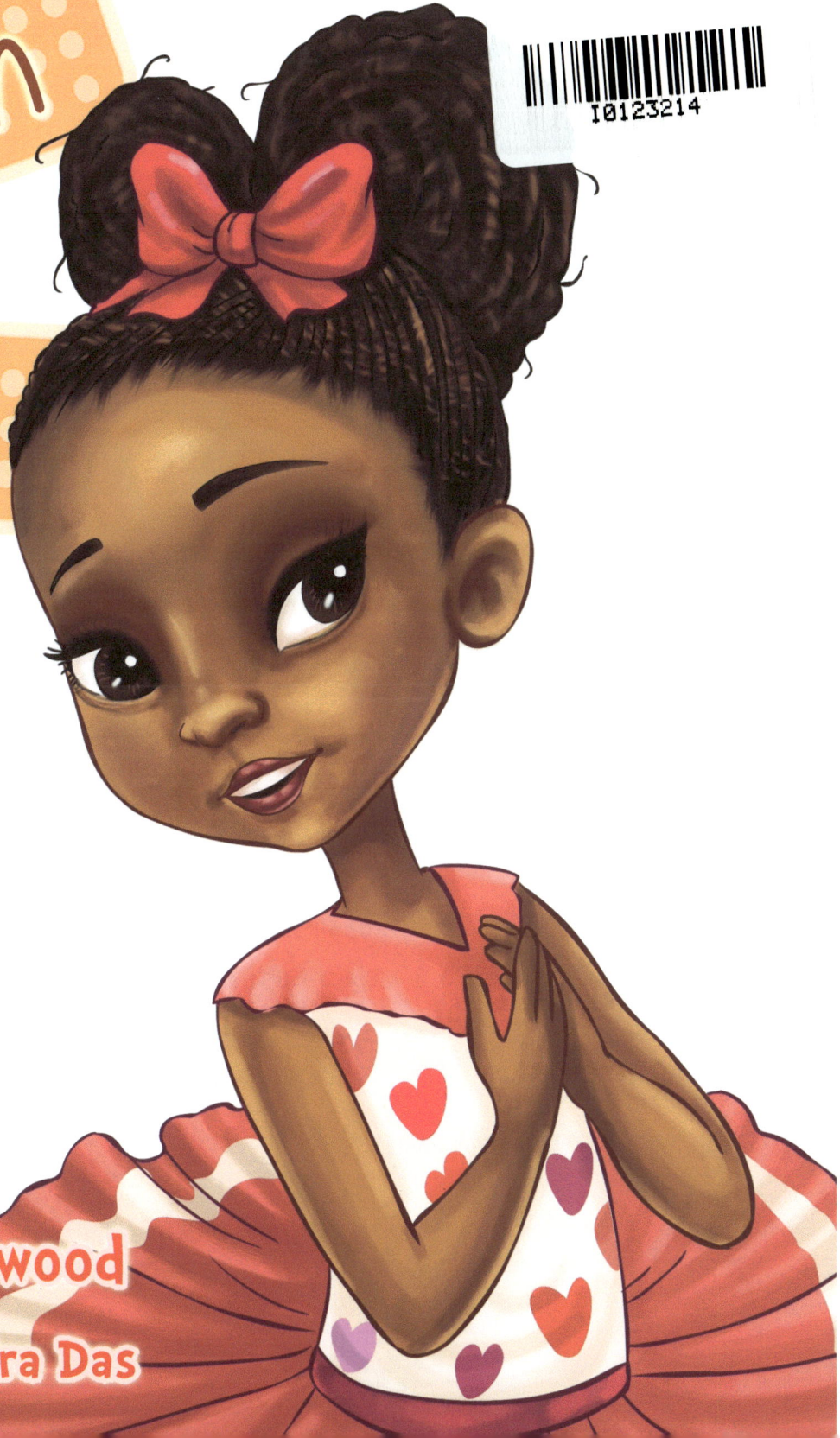

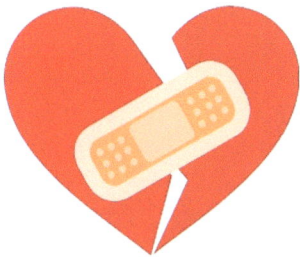

By: A'Quita Fullwood

Illustrated By: Abira Das

Printed in the United States of America.
First Printing, 2018
Cover Design and Illustrations by Abira Das
Edited by Val Pugh–Love
ISBN: 978–0–692–10674–7
A 'Quita's Heart, LLC
Shreveport, LA 71107
www.amazon.com/author/aquitafullwood

Dedication

To God, my parents, my brothers, my family, my school, the doctors and staff of Ochsner Medical Center in Baton Rouge, LA, and my cardiologist, Dr. Jones...

"Mom! Mom! May I please go outside?"
I asked as I quickly ran into Mom's room.

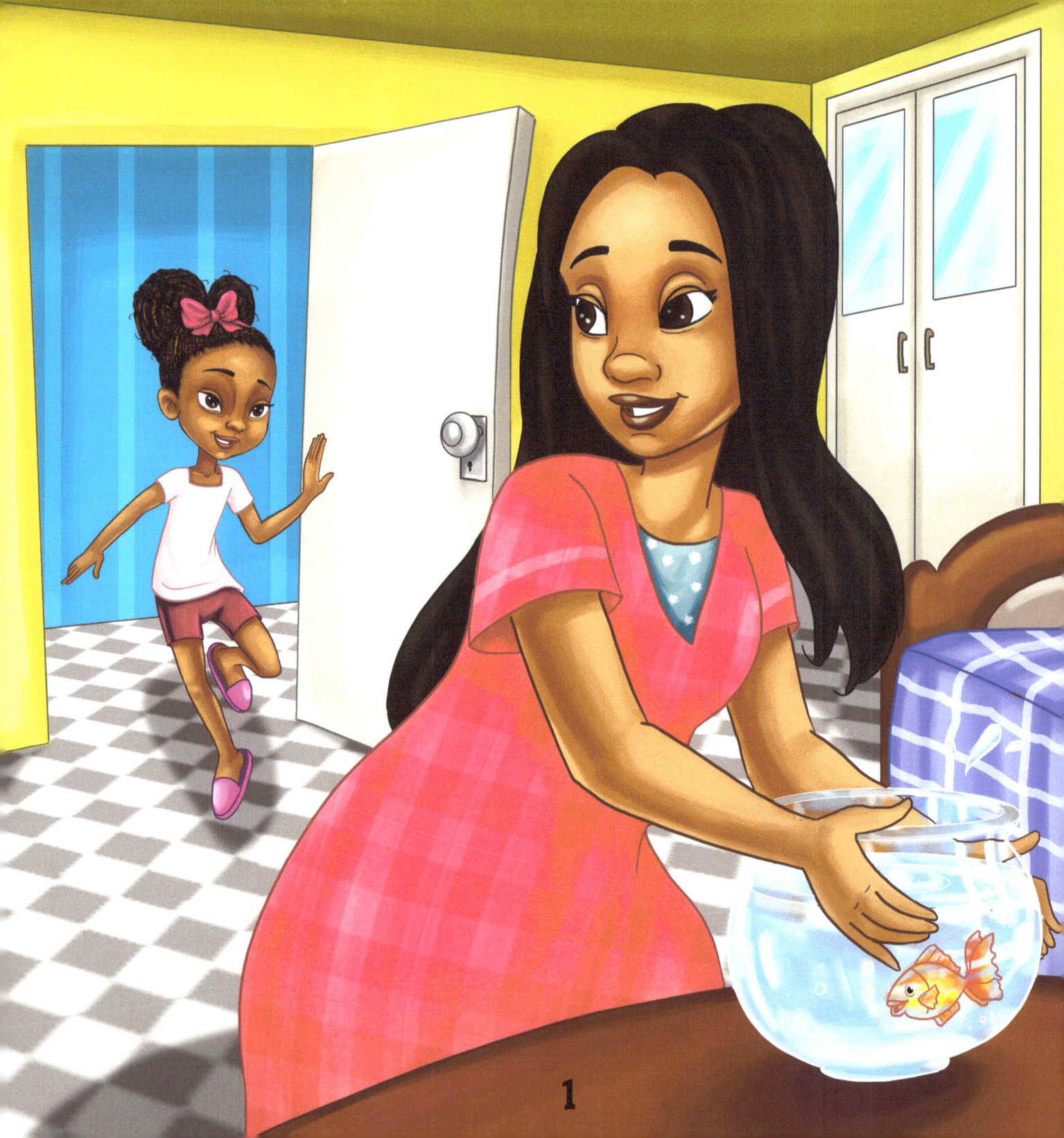

"Have you cleaned your room?"
"Yes, ma'am!" I replied with glee.
"Sure, Ladybug," she said.

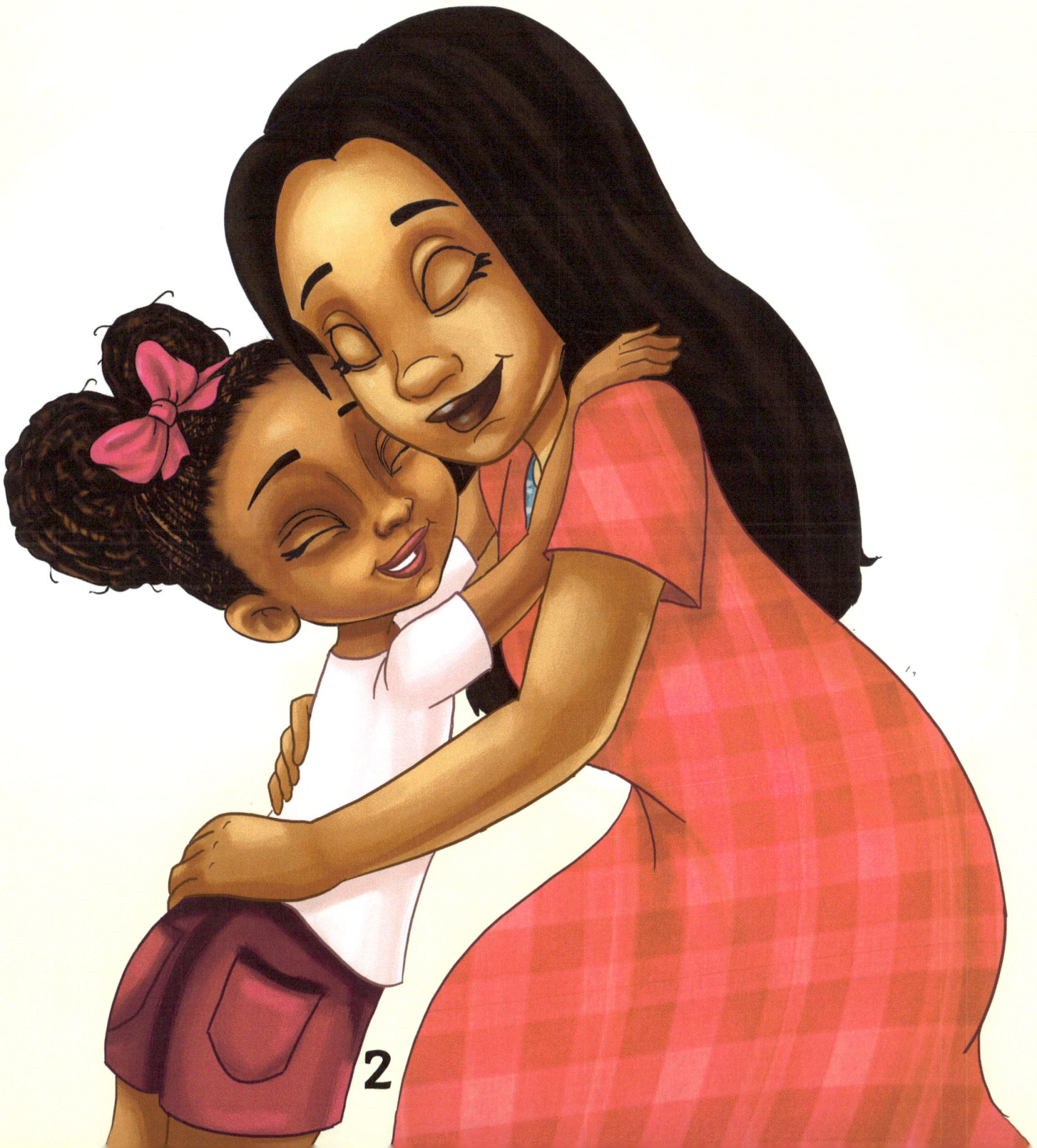

2

In a flash, I ran to my room, put on my shoes, and headed outside to enjoy the day.

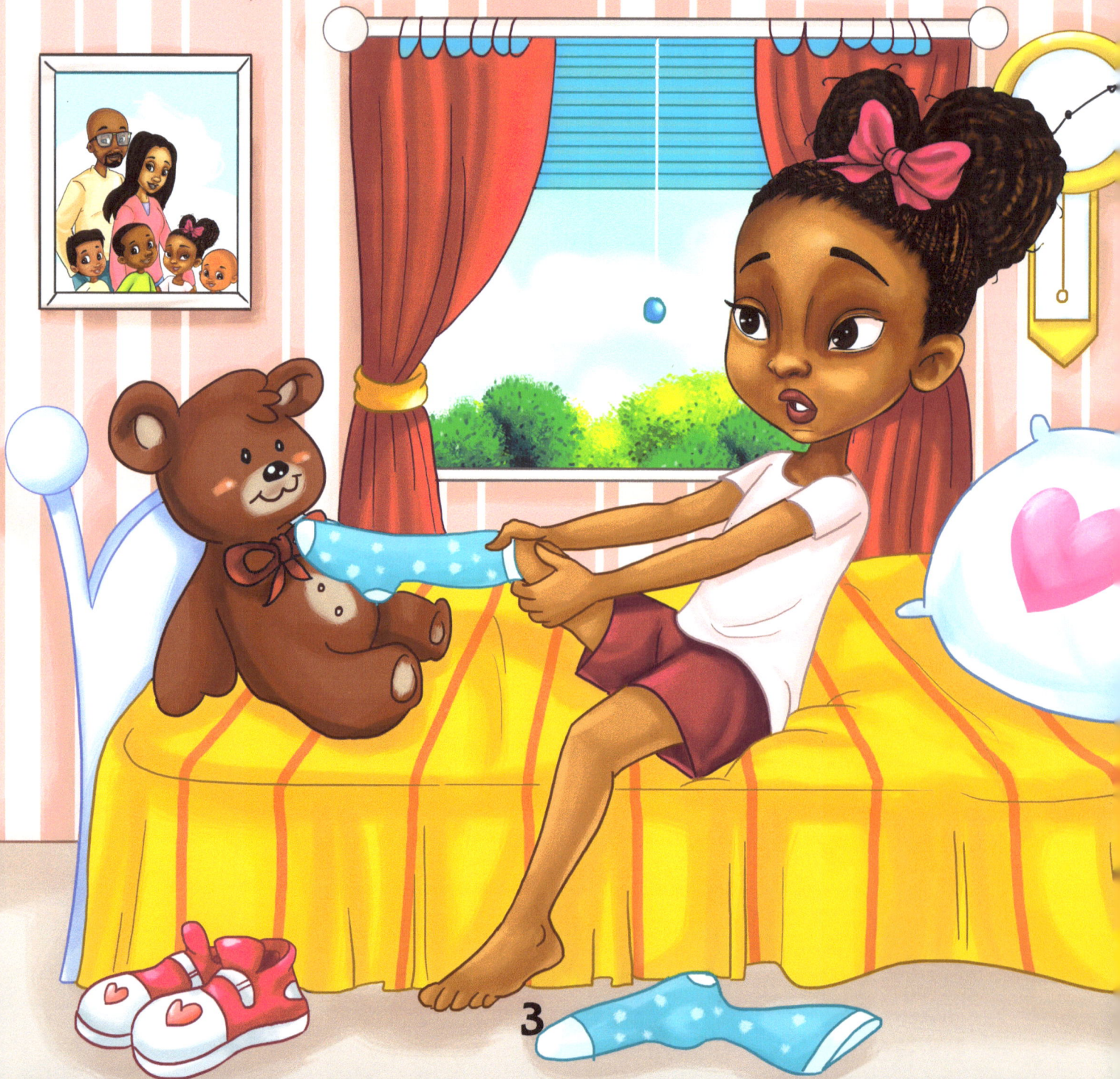

3

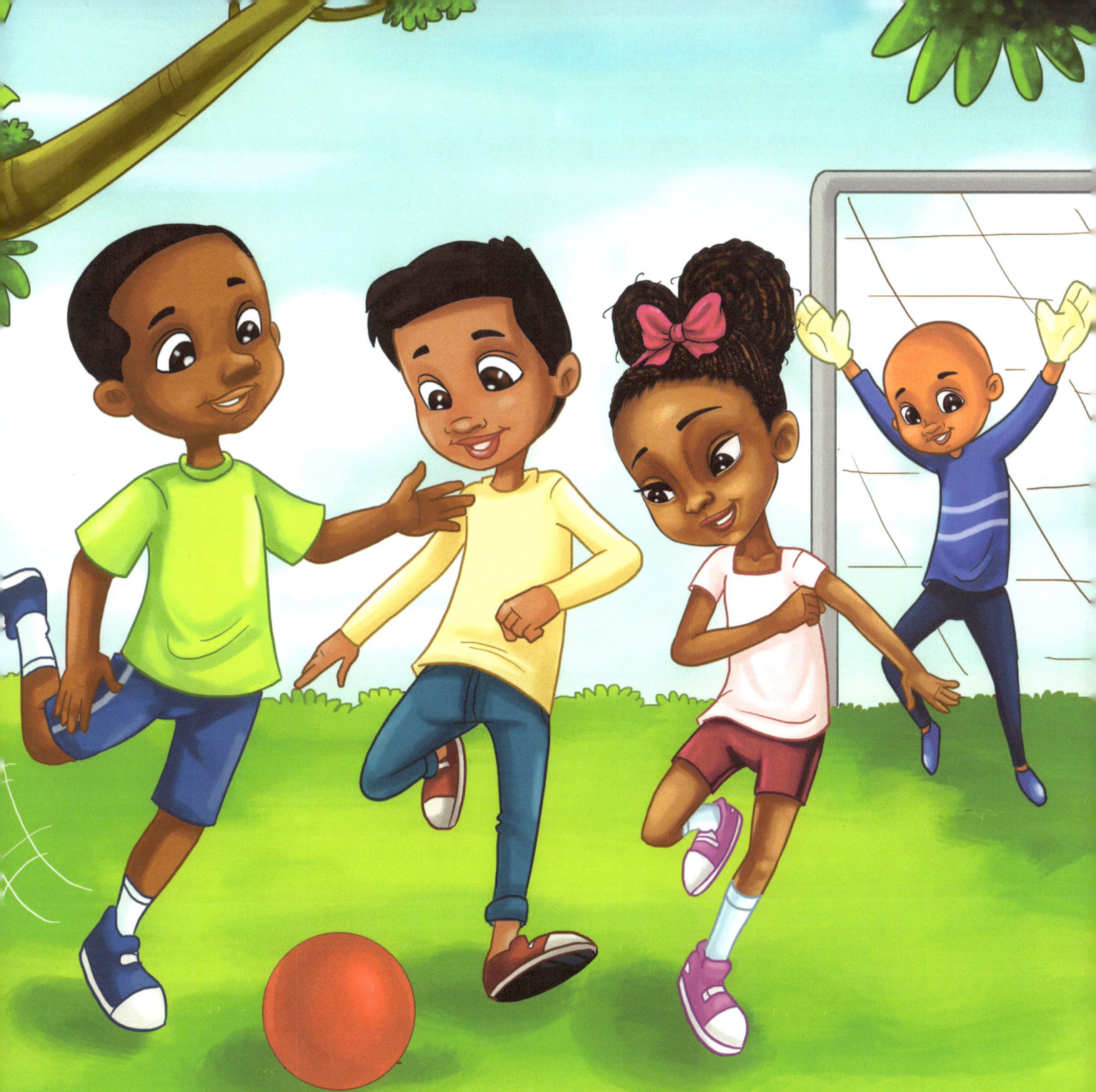

When I got to the backyard,
I saw my brothers running and playing.
I gladly joined their game.

We were running and kicking the ball
everywhere when I suddenly
I began to feel pain and
more pain in my chest.

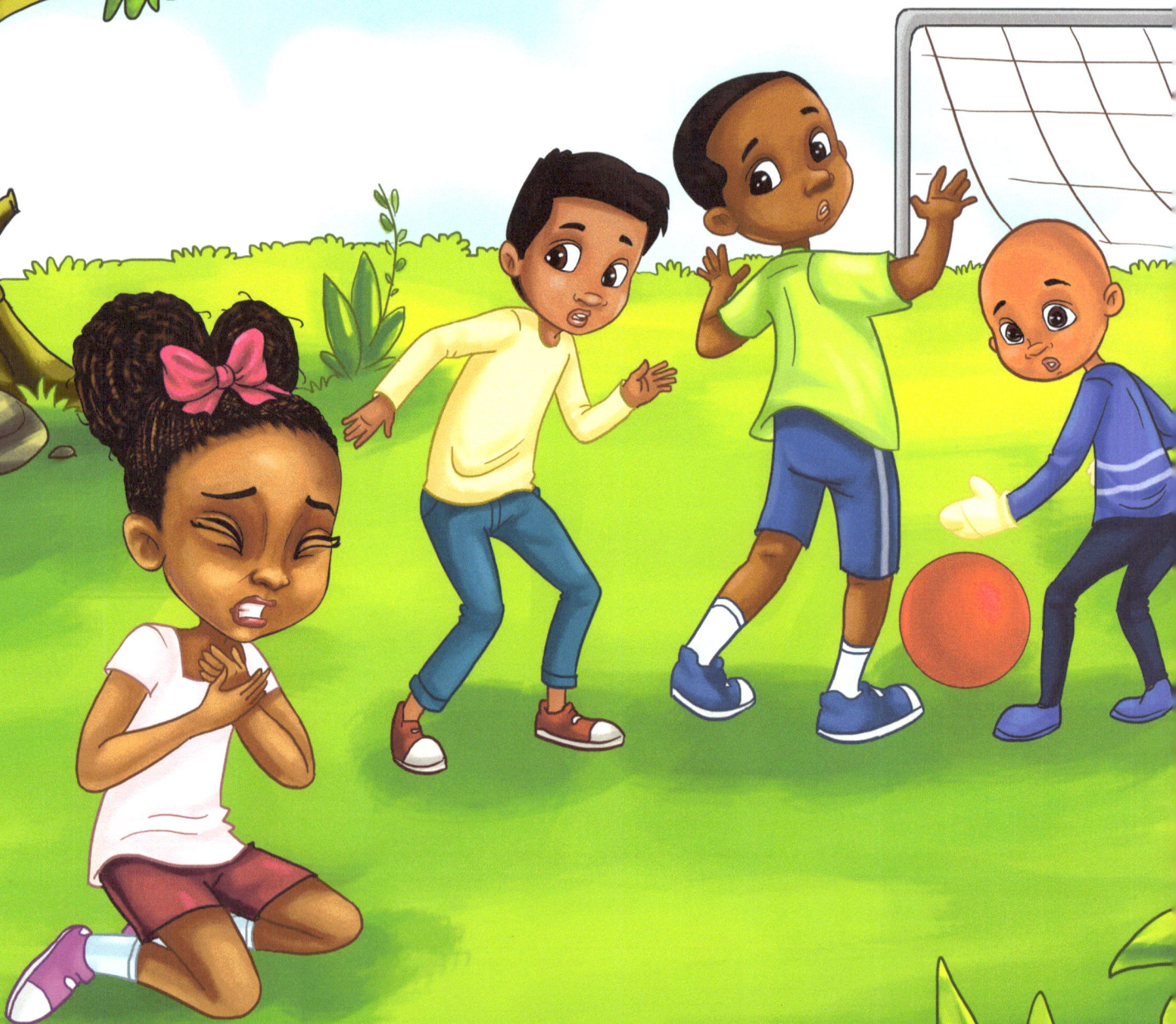

I fell to the ground and yelled to my brothers, "Go get mom!" I knew she would handle this the best. I remember seeing her run out of the house to my side. Everything after that is a blur.

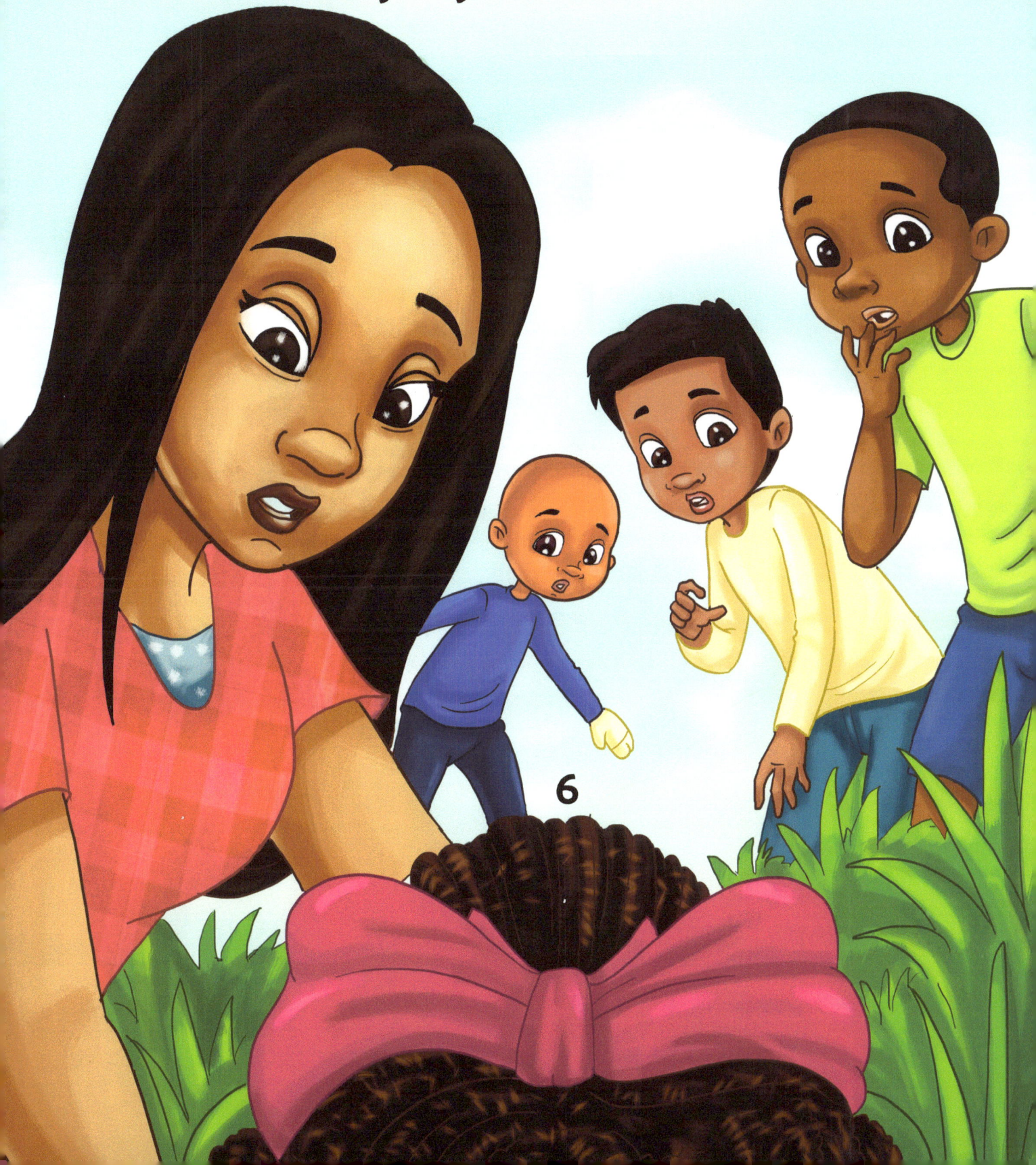

6

Several days later, I woke up to a lot of machines attached to my chest and head. When I looked to my left, I saw my mom and dad standng near my hospital bed.

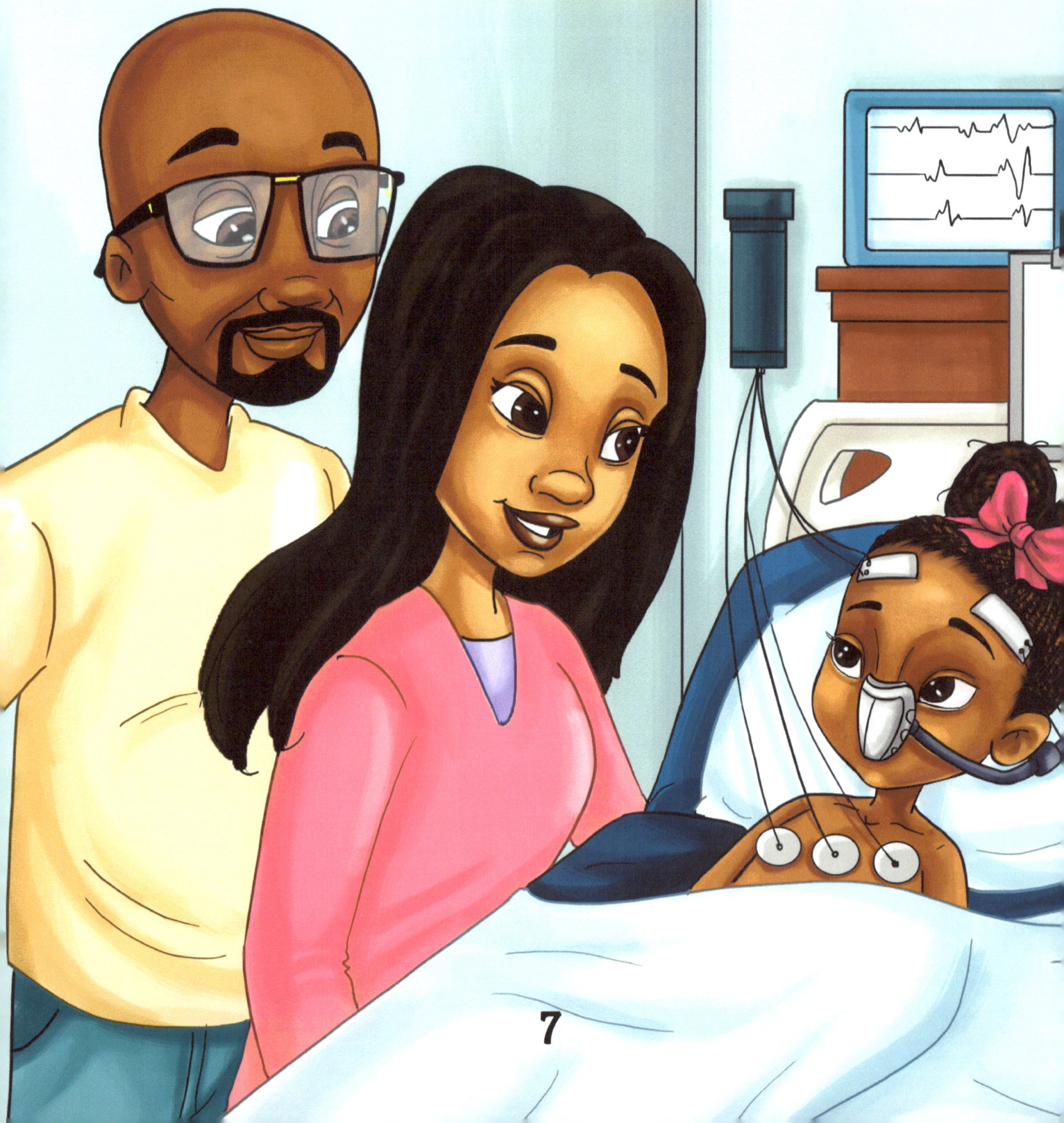

"How do you feel?" Dad asked.
"Like a bus hit me."
Mom shook her head in dismay and explained to me that
my heart is broken and special
doctors will have to fix it.

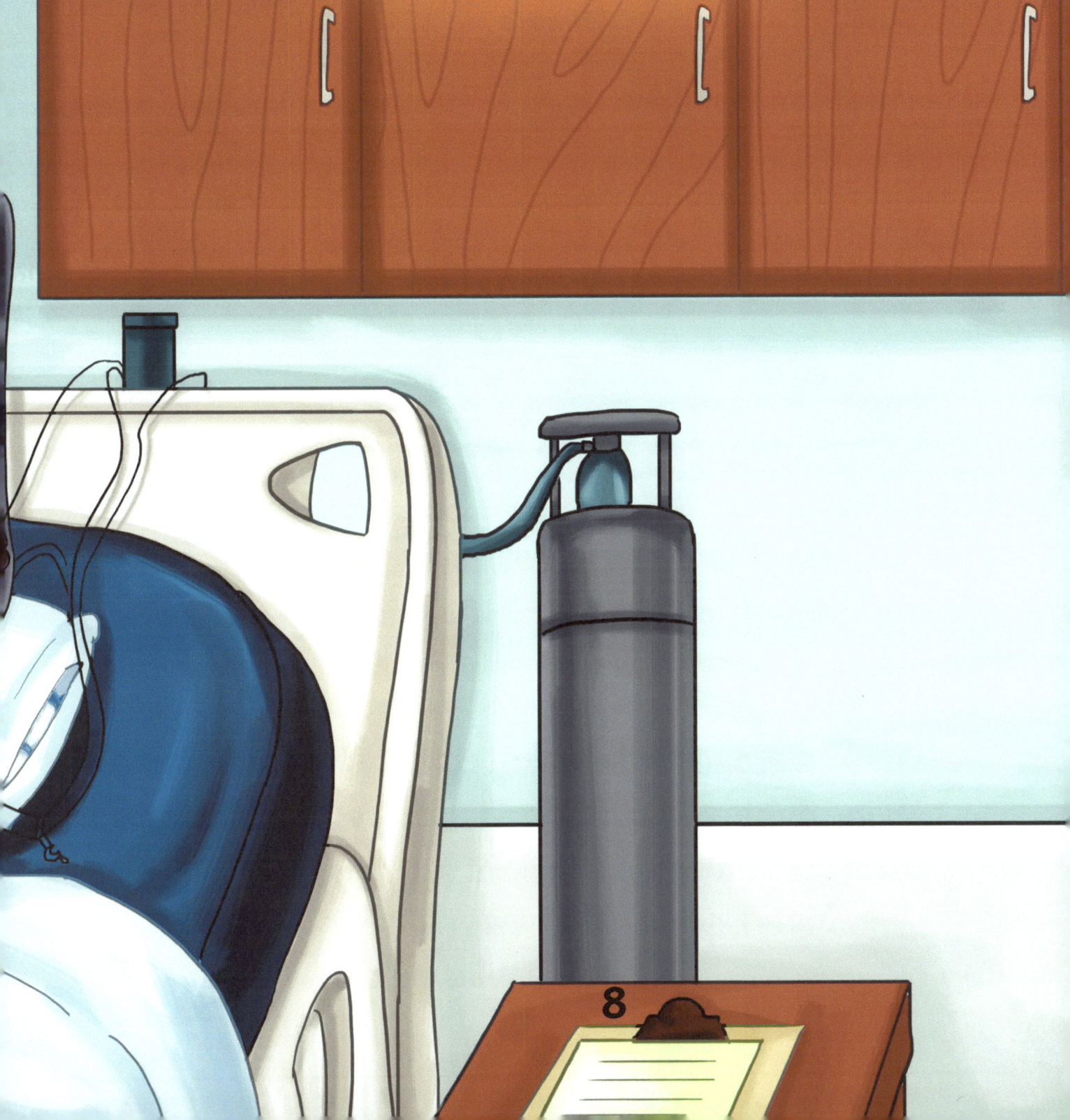

8

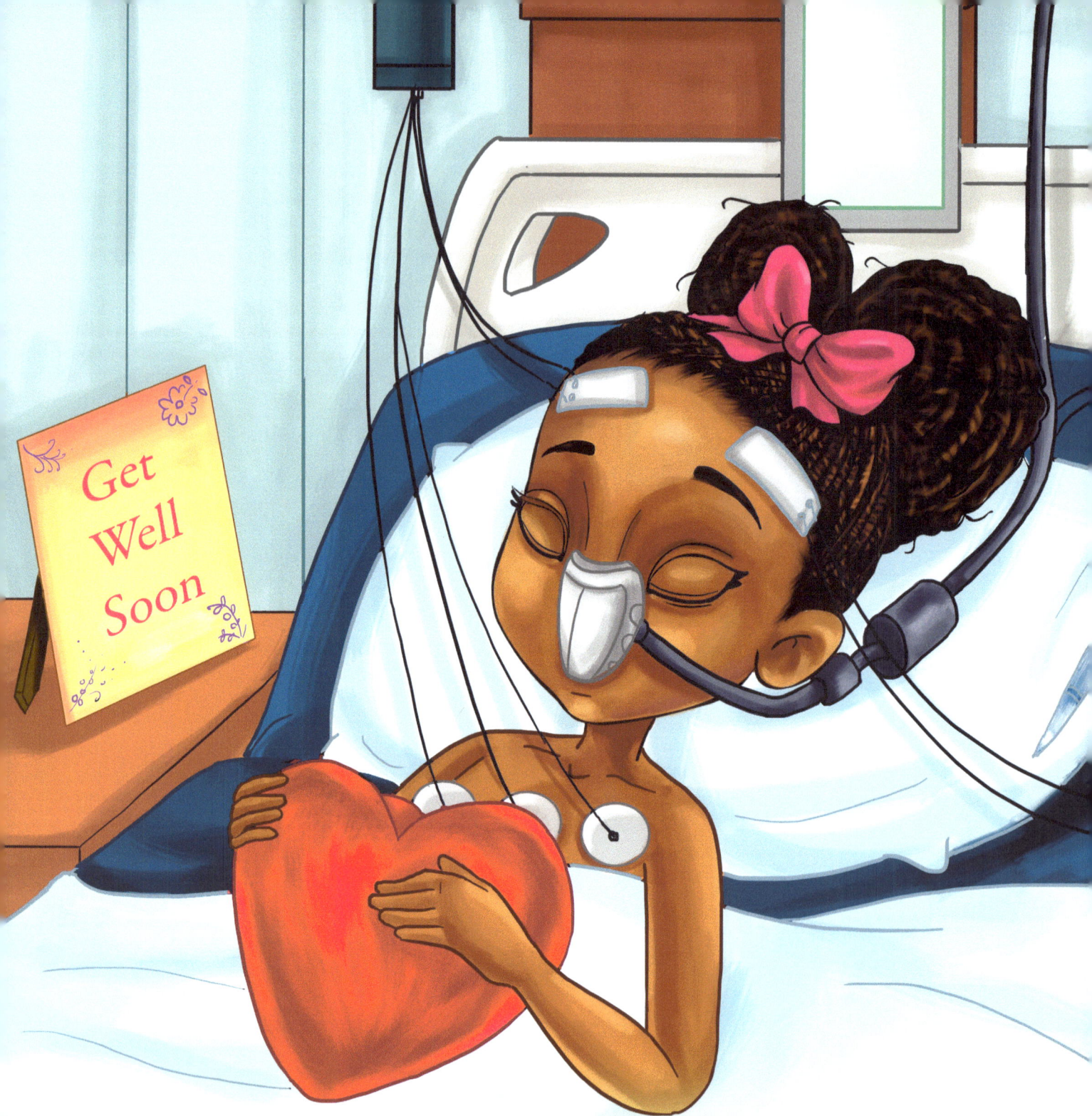

I looked around with a very confused face. "I was just playing outside with my brothers. How did this happen?" "Just get some rest. You have surgery in the morning," Mom replied. The news didn't frighten me, but it did make me cry.

I woke up early the next morning to get ready for my big day.
Guess what... All my family was there to see me away!

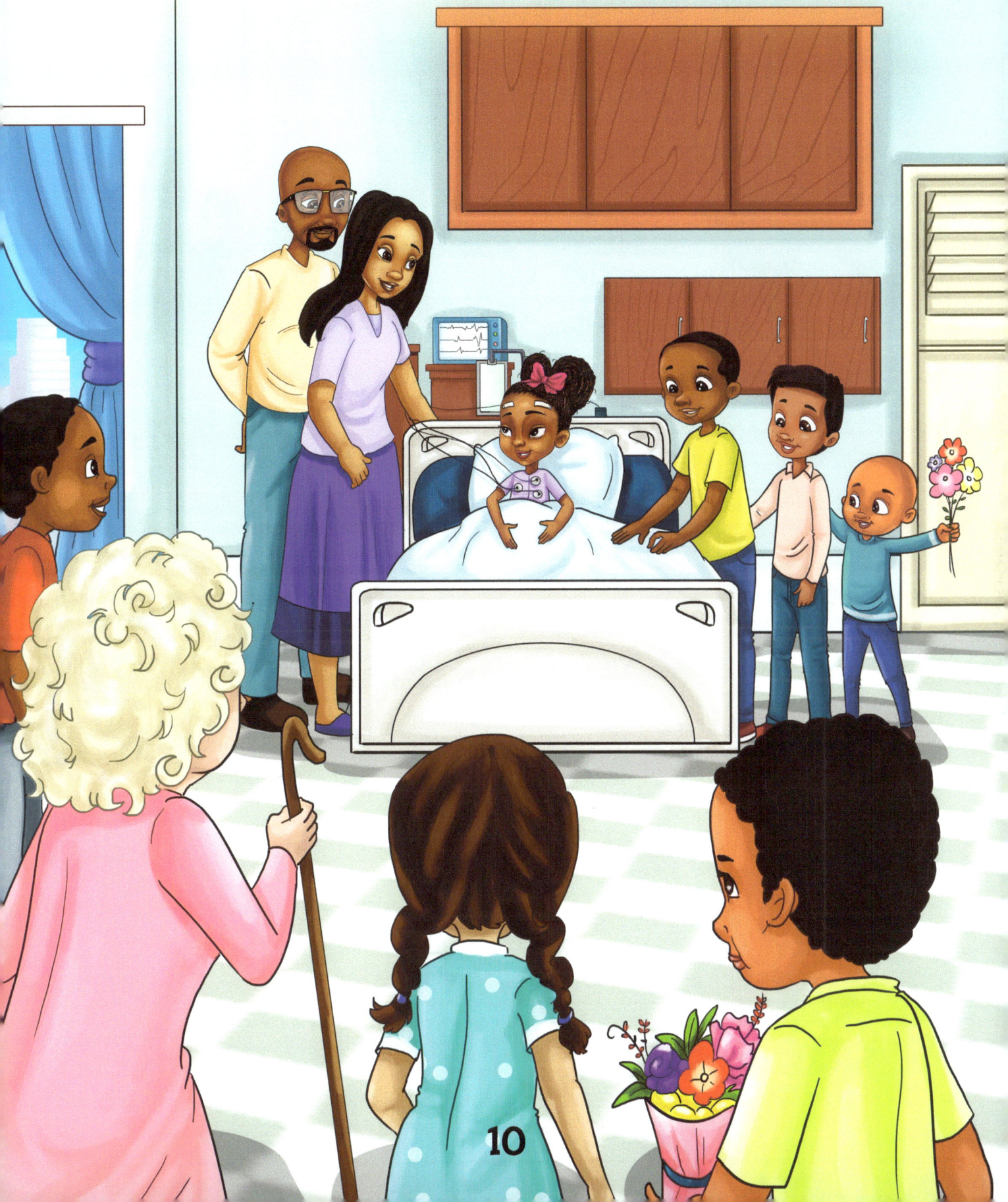

The surgery lasted over ten hours! I slept the entire time, but God was right in the room. He really helped me survive. When I woke up, I was back in my hospital room with all my family by my side. This time, I couldn't help but to cry.

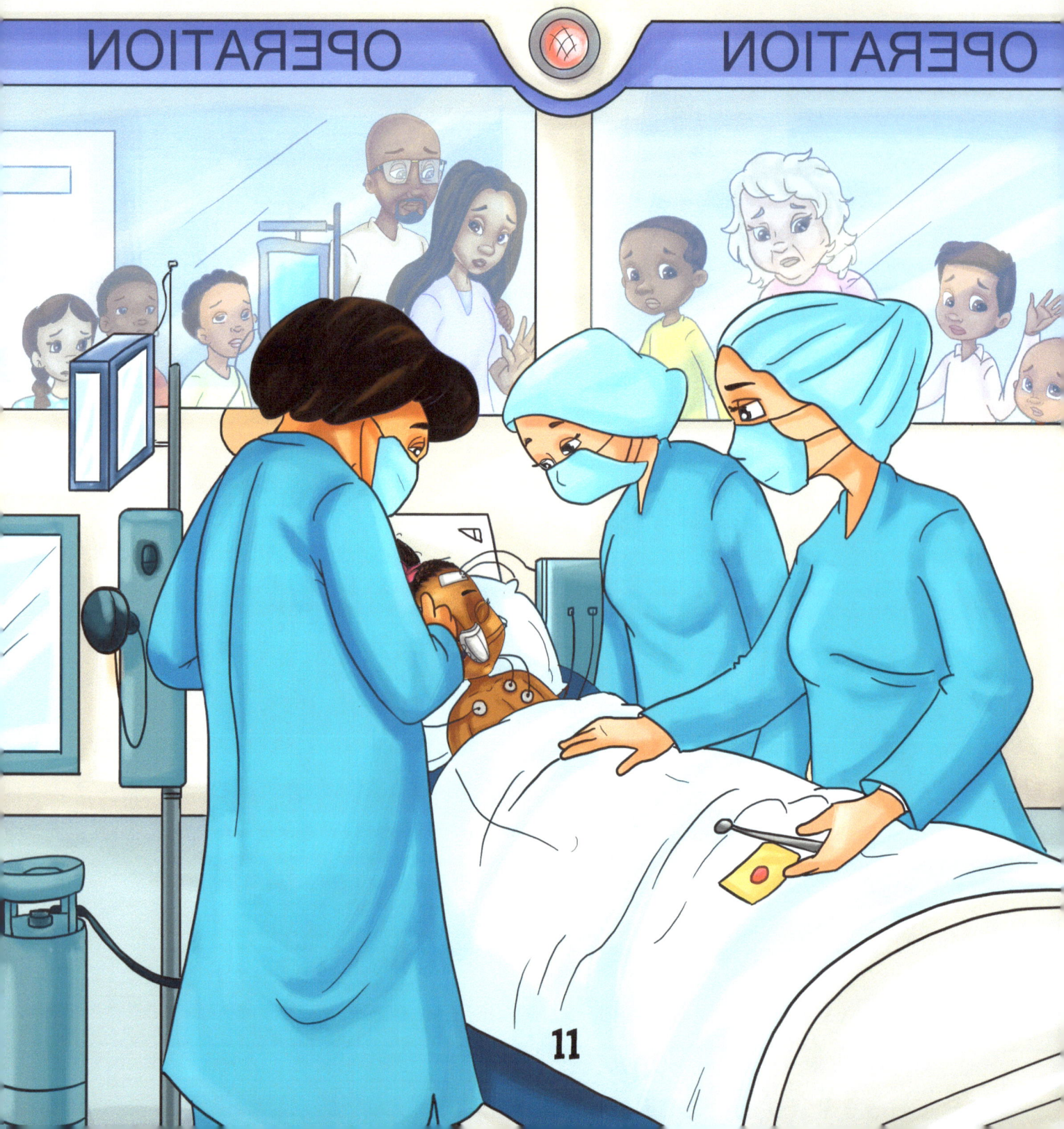

My first night home was the hardest for me. Again, I asked my mom, "What really happened to me?" She looked at me with a smile and said, "It's all over now."

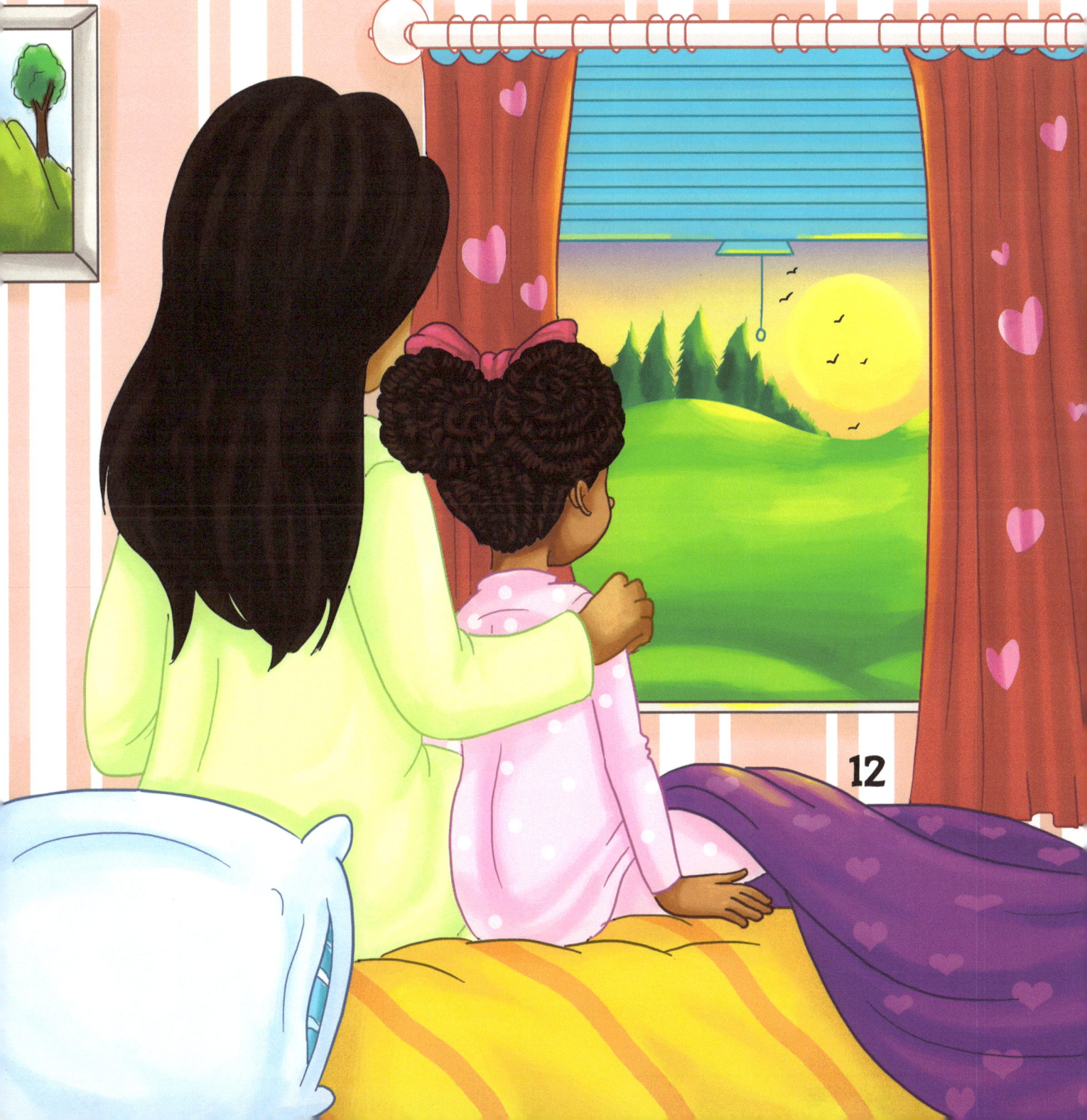

12

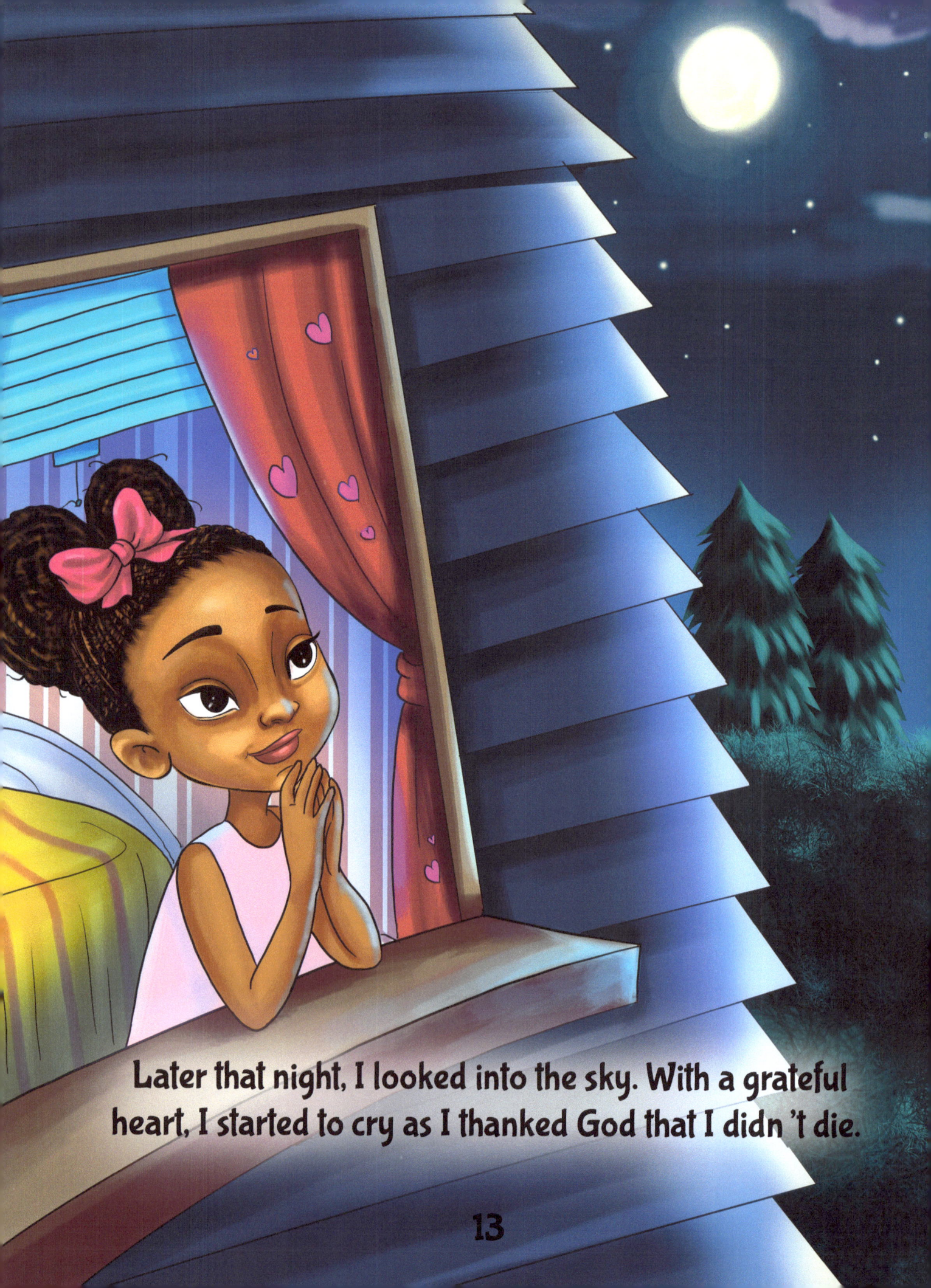

Later that night, I looked into the sky. With a grateful heart, I started to cry as I thanked God that I didn't die.

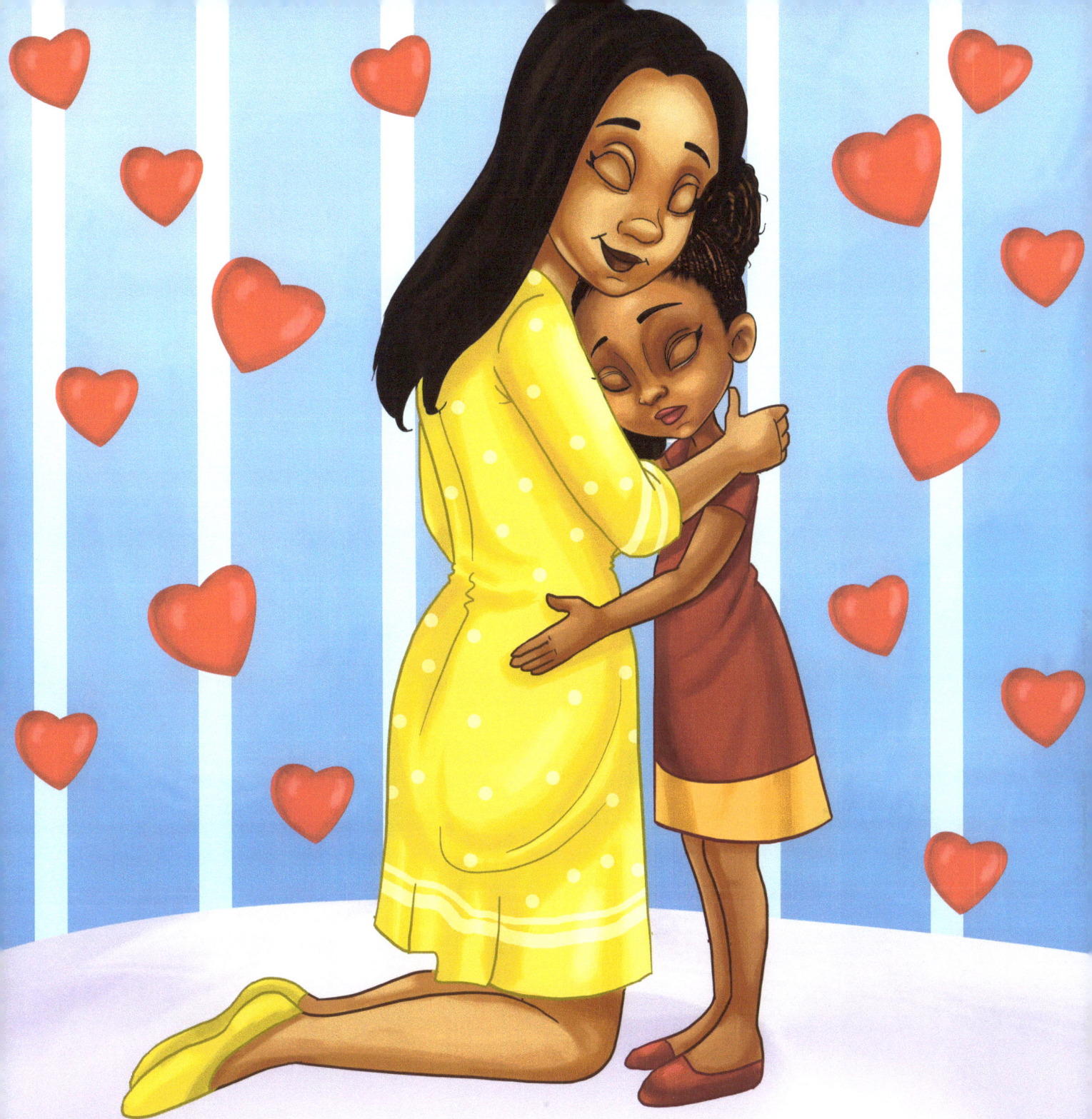

The next morning, I was talking to my mom.
I told her that I was very blessed.
She looked into my eyes and said,
"Yes, God is the best."

14

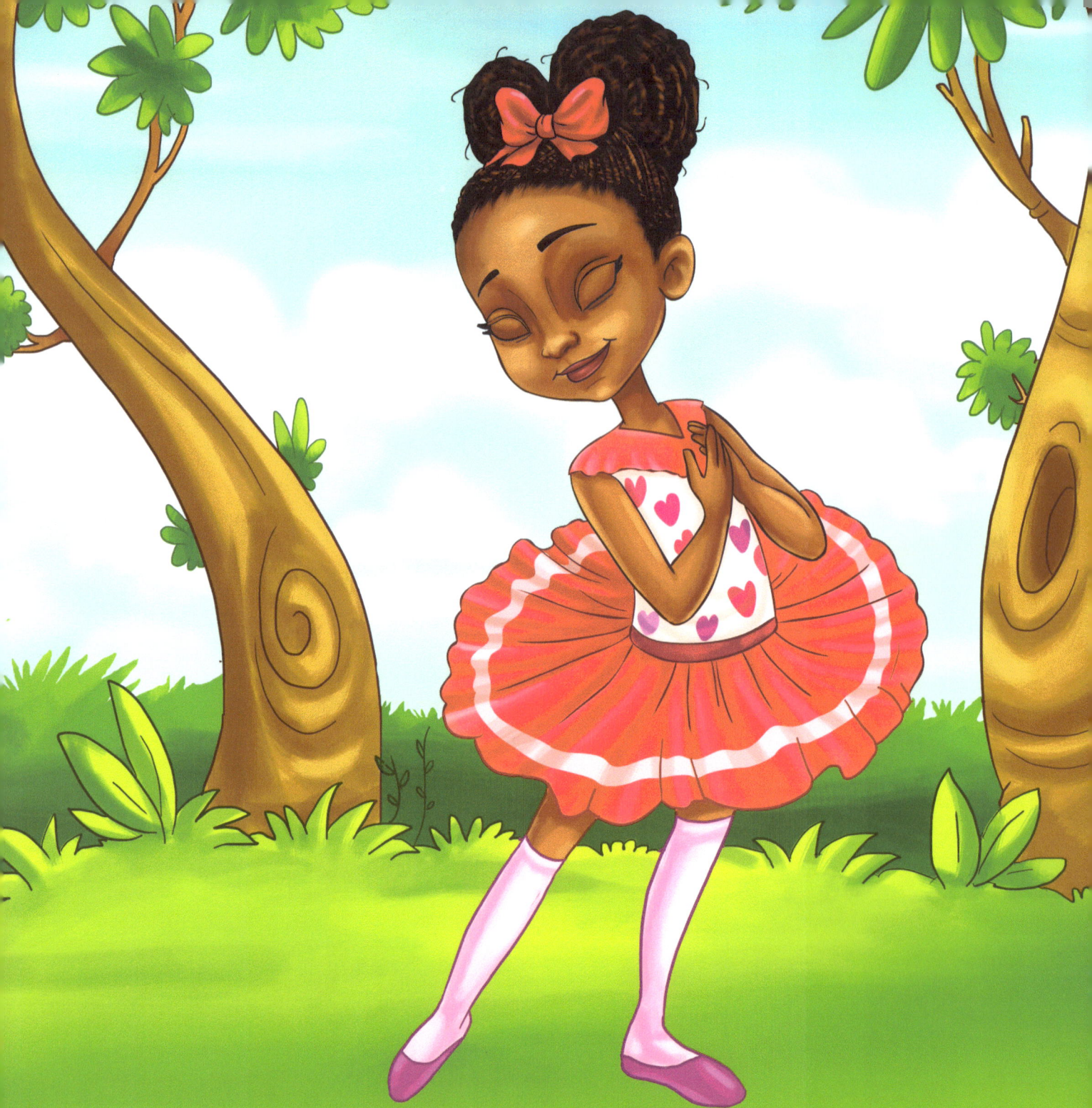

Now everywhere I go, I will tell every one I know about the man who thought enough of me to make my heart so complete. I am forever grateful...

My Hospital Stay

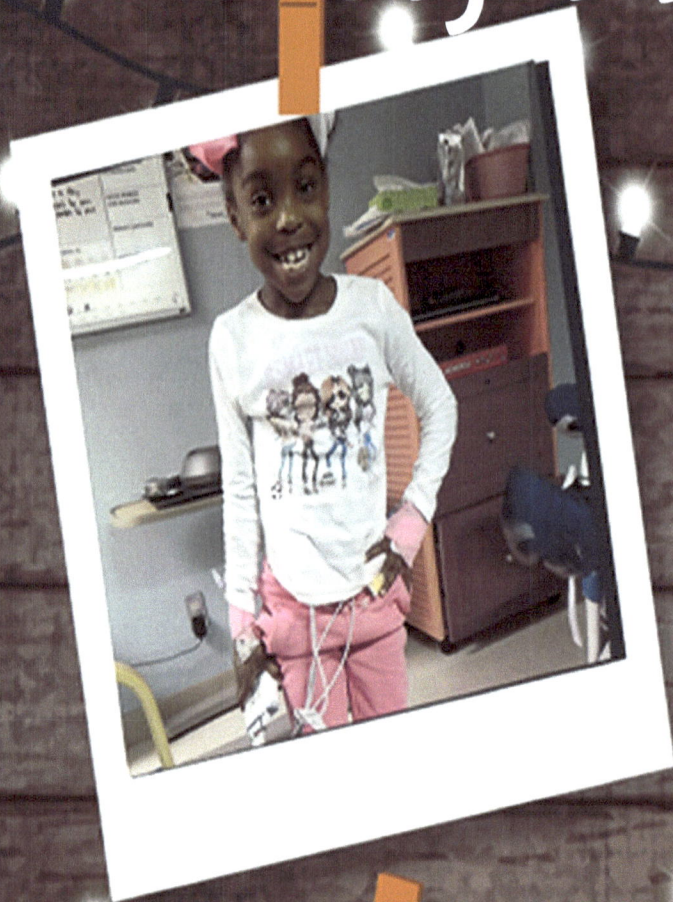

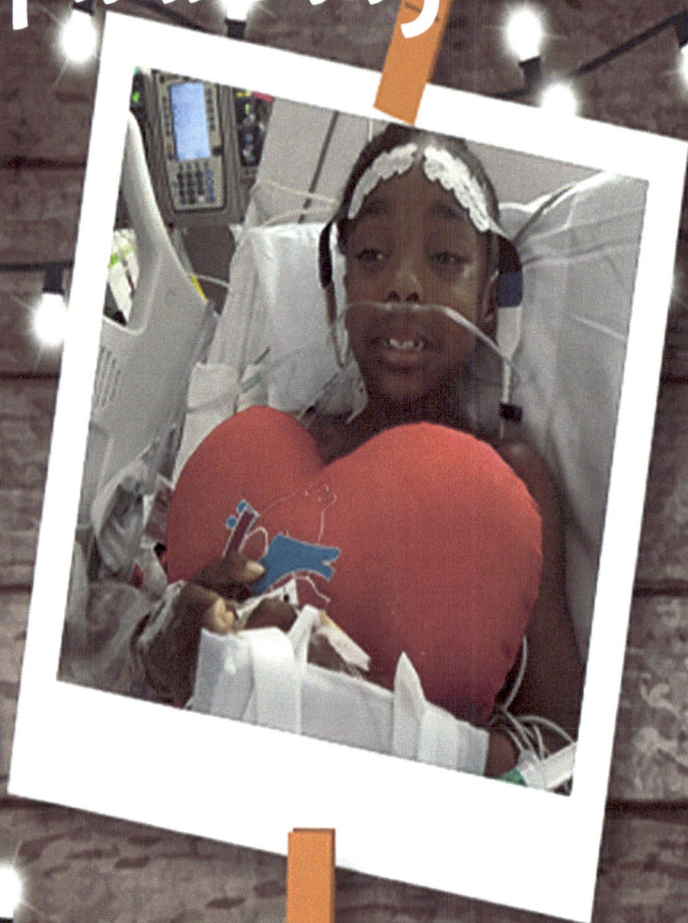

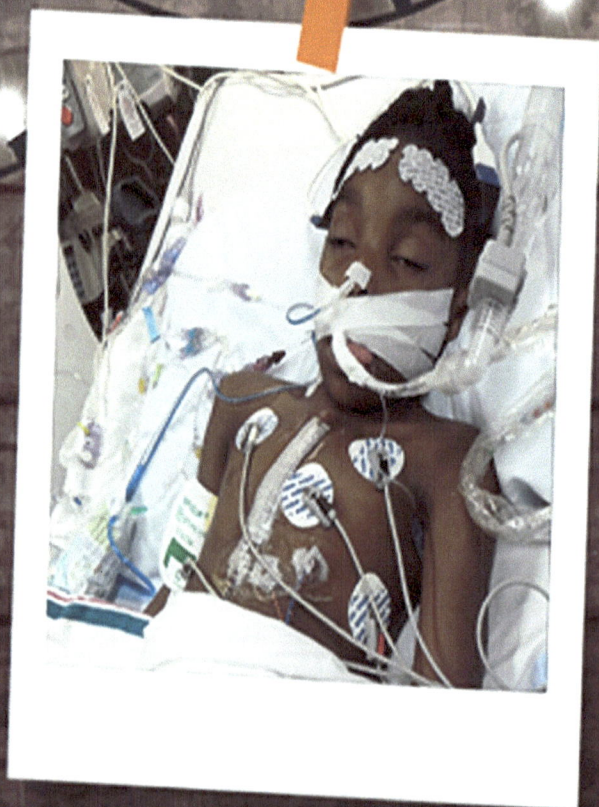

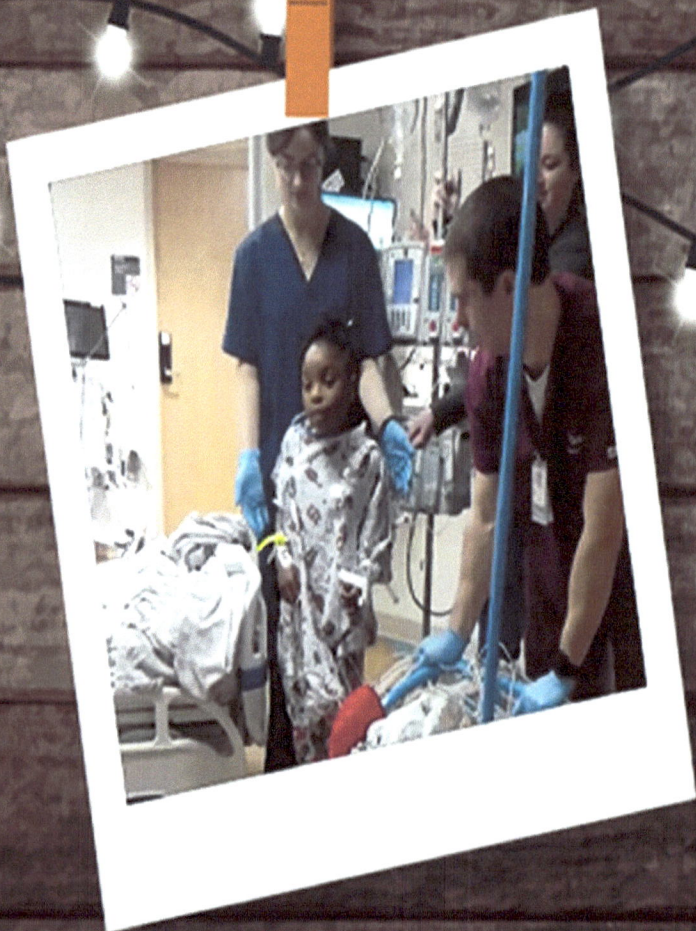

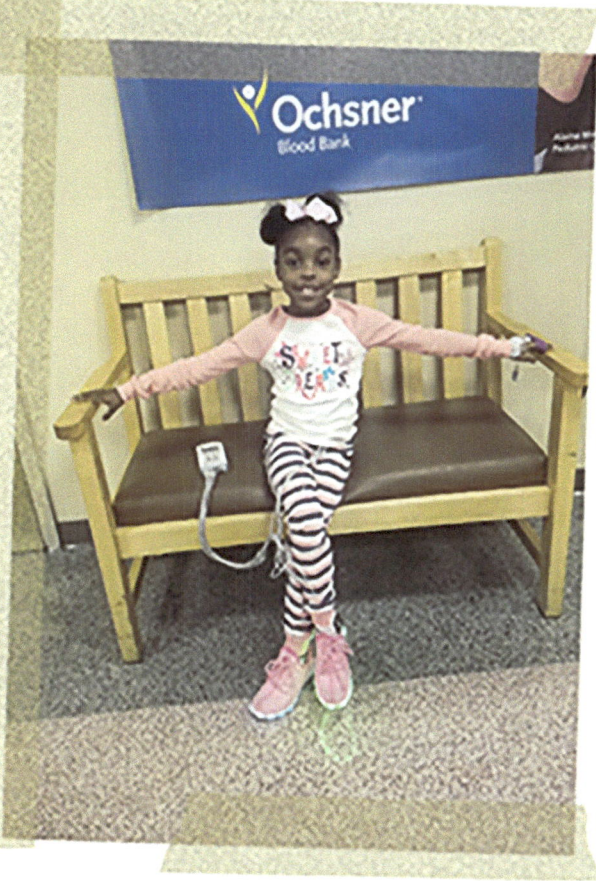

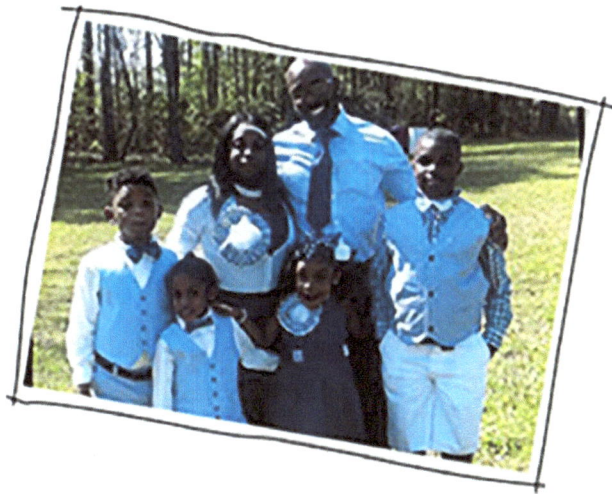

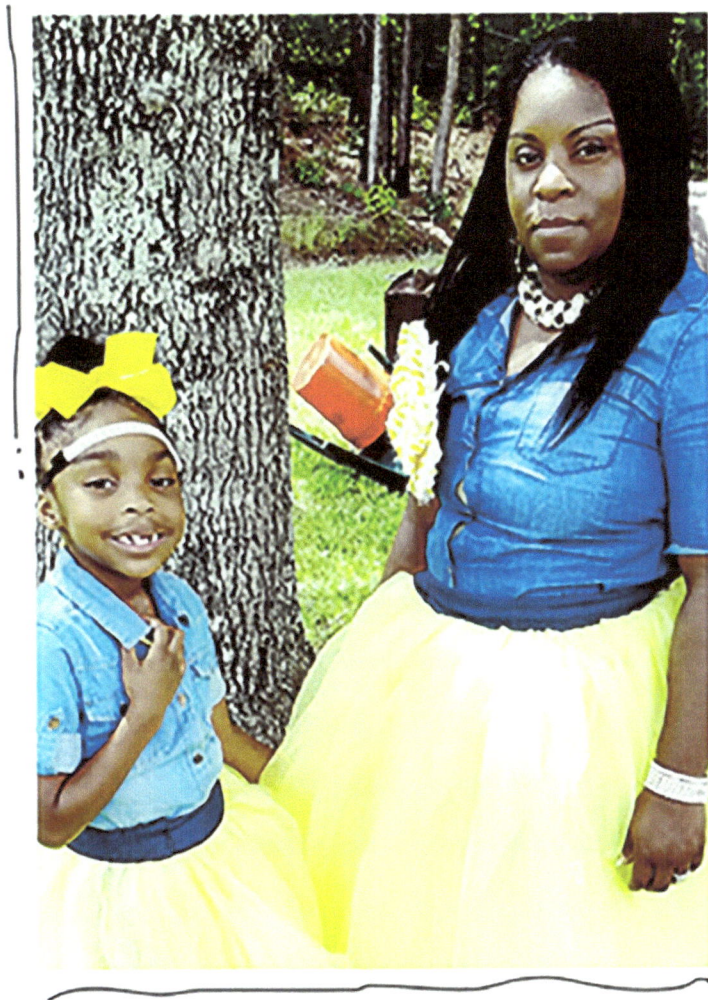

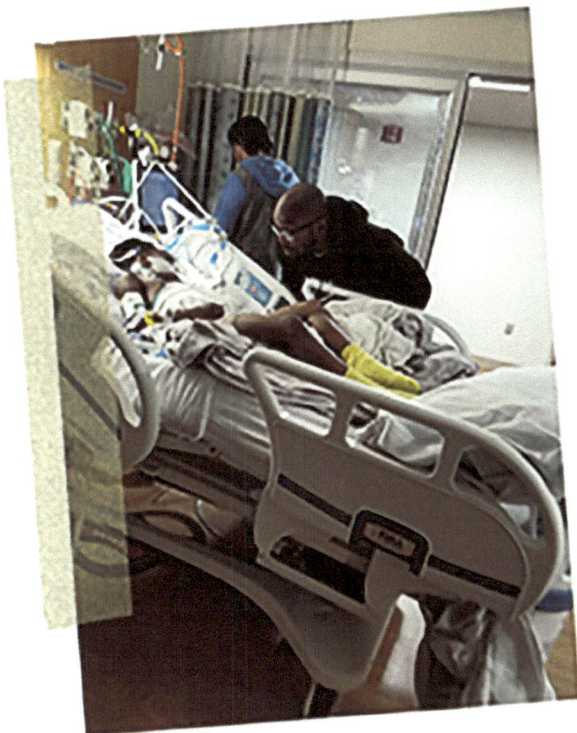

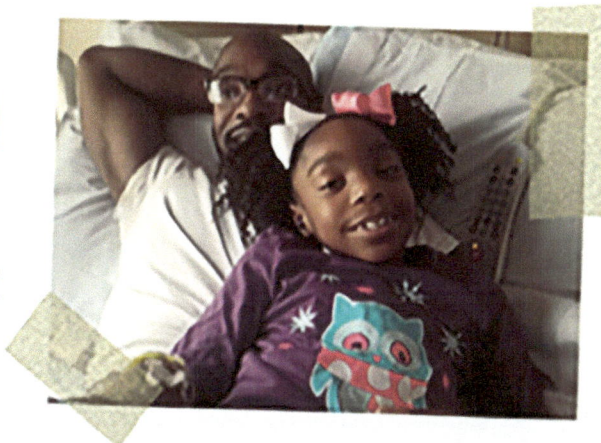

My Family & Me

www.ingramcontent.com/pod-product-compliance
Lightning Source LLC
Chambersburg PA
CBHW060856270326
41934CB00002B/160